D1722881

Disclaimer

This book is intended to help people become better informed medical consumers. The information in this book is intended to supplement, not replace, the medical advice of a trained health care professional. No mention or description of uses of drugs listed herein should be construed as an endorsement of those uses or drugs. Only a physician can prescribe drugs and their precise dosages. All matters regarding your health require medical supervision. The authors and publisher disclaim any liability arising directly or indirectly from use of this book.

Notice of rights

Trademarks

Many of the designations used by manufacturers and sellers to distinguish their products are claimed as trademarks. Where those designations appear in this book, and the publisher was aware of a trademark claim, the designations appear as requested by the owner of the trademark. All other product names and services identified throughout this book are used in editorial fashion only and for the benefit of such companies with no intention of infringement of the trademark. No such use, or the use of any trade name, is intended to convey endorsement or other affiliation with this book.

Table of Contents

Your feedback is invaluable to us

If you recently bought this book, we would love to hear from you! You can do this by writing a review on amazon (or the online store where you purchased this book) about your last purchase! As part of our continual service improvement process, we love to hear real client experiences and feedback.

How does it work?
To post a review on Amazon, just log in to your account and click on the Create Your Own Review button (under Customer Reviews) of the relevant product page. You can find examples of product reviews in Amazon. If you purchased from another online store, simply follow their procedures.

Why use this book?

Everyone should ask questions when getting a prescription. This is especially important when your doctor or other health care professional prescribes you Pentobarbital Sodium.

What should you ask?

Your health depends on good communication, but which questions to ask your doctor? Having the right questions is the answer.

Asking questions and providing information to your doctor and other care providers can improve your care. Talking with your doctor builds trust and leads to better satisfaction, quality, safety and results.

Asking questions is key to good communication with your doctor. If you do not ask questions, he or she may assume you already know the answer or that you do not want more information. Do not wait for the doctor to raise a specific question or subject; he or she may not know it is important to you. Be proactive. Ask questions.

Effective health care is a team effort. You are part of this team and play an important role. One of the best ways to communicate with your doctor and health care team is by asking questions. Since time is limited when you have your medical appointments, you will feel less rushed when you prepare your questions before your appointment.

Your doctor wants your questions. Doctors know a lot about a lot of things, but they do not always know everything about you, what you want to know or what is best for you.

Your questions give your doctor and health care professionals important information about you, like your most important health care concerns.

That is why they need you to speak up.

How to use this book?

When you meet with your doctor or other members of your health care team, you will hear a lot of information. It helps to think ahead of time of the things you want to know and to highlight the questions in this book you want to ask and take this book with you to your appointments.

This book contains questions you may want to ask your doctor. You should use the questions that fit your situation, and skip those that do not apply.

This book offers many ways that you can ask questions and get your health care needs met. With this book you will have numerous simple questions that can help you take better care of yourself, feel better, and get the right care at the right time.

Doctors and medical professionals want to know your questions to help them take better care of you and offer advice to get your most pressing questions answered.

Be prepared for your next medical appointment. Take this book with you if you are getting a checkup, want to discuss a problem or health condition, are getting a prescription, or talk about a medical test or surgery and be sure to write down the answers your health care professional provides for you in this book.

Whatever the reason for your appointment, it is important to be prepared.

Take charge of your health. Ask your health care providers questions and learn about the Pentobarbital Sodium medicine you take.

BEGINNING OF THE QUESTION CHAPTERS:

CHAPTER #1: WHO:

INTENT: Who benefits from Pentobarbital Sodium (Is this right for me.)

1. If I am unable to comply with the treatment regimen, who else can administer Pentobarbital Sodium medication?

Notes:

2. Is _____ normal to get after only been taking the Pentobarbital Sodium medication for a few days?

Notes:

3. Does my plan cover my Pentobarbital Sodium prescription drugs?

Notes:

4. Are there any side effects associated with this Pentobarbital Sodium medication that I should know about?

Notes:

5. Is there a possibility of reaction to Pentobarbital Sodium medications?

Notes:

6. Who typically uses Pentobarbital Sodium prescription drugs, and where do they get them?

Notes:

7. Who is validating my Pentobarbital Sodium prescription drugs to make sure I am taking the correct pills?

Notes:

8. What do each of these Pentobarbital Sodium prescription medications have in common?

Notes:

9. Who is most susceptible to Pentobarbital Sodium prescription drug abuse?

Notes:

10. Are the supplements I take worthwhile?

Notes:

11. I Googled my symptoms and read this. Is it accurate?

Notes:

12. Are any medications I am taking dangerous for my stage of this disease?

Notes:

13. Is there any form of exercise or medication you can recommend to enhance the effects of Pentobarbital Sodium?

Notes:

14. How do you help someone who has a Pentobarbital Sodium prescription drugs addiction?

Notes:

15. Can Canadian drug pharmacies mail my Pentobarbital Sodium prescription drugs and medications to me?

Notes:

16. Who can join a Medicare Pentobarbital Sodium prescription drug plan?

Notes:

17. Are there any supplements or Pentobarbital Sodium medications?

Notes:

18. Who gets to see the Pentobarbital Sodium prescription drug information submitted in my patient medical questionnaire?

Notes:

19. What if I am currently without prescription drug coverage?

Notes:

20. Who is qualified to receive Pentobarbital Sodium prescription drug help?

Notes:

21. If the pharmacist offers me a different brand of the same Pentobarbital Sodium-like medicine - is it ok to take it?

Notes:

22. Are side effects from Pentobarbital Sodium medications the same in males and females?

Notes:

23. Are there any co-pays for medical treatments, hospitalization or Pentobarbital Sodium prescription drugs?

Notes:

24. Can you help me with finding the money to purchase doctor visits and also Pentobarbital Sodium prescriptions medication?

Notes:

25. How do you prevent re-admission in case I forget to take my Pentobarbital Sodium prescription medications. How do you help those who have problems following suggestions regarding eating habits, smoking, drinking, and taking drugs..?

Notes:

26. Is Pentobarbital Sodium medication a substitute for therapy?

Notes:

27. Does Medicaid cover Pentobarbital Sodium prescription medications?

Notes:

28. Who makes this Pentobarbital Sodium medication?

Notes:

29. Can my baby get harmed by my Pentobarbital Sodium prescription drug use?

Notes:

30. Will Pentobarbital Sodium cause me to test positive for various substances in a urine drug test?

Notes:

31. What treatments, therapies and medications are recommended or available for my condition?

Notes:

32. What are the Pentobarbital Sodium prescription drug prices?

Notes:

33. When in care who is responsible for the MAR (Medication Administration Records), who can put information on to it and make changes?

Notes:

34. Can Pentobarbital Sodium be mixed with other medications, dietary supplements, or alcohol?

Notes:

35. Is there anything I should do to help prevent my health issue?

Notes:

36. How can a wholesome mud-bath help my condition, and what is the effect on my Pentobarbital Sodium prescription drugs?

Notes:

37. Do enzymes interfere with Pentobarbital Sodium prescription drugs?

Notes:

38. Who can I contact if I want to meet with a specialist for long-term Pentobarbital Sodium

medication management on an ongoing basis?

Notes:

39. If I could possibly reduce the number of prescription drugs besides Pentobarbital Sodium I have to take for various conditions and feel a lot better by taking a single substance, would you look into it?

Notes:

40. Can people be guilty of DUI if they are driving under the influence of Pentobarbital Sodium prescription medications?

Notes:

41. What does using a prescription drug Off-label mean?

Notes:

42. Has there been any follow up of those who have stopped taking Pentobarbital Sodium medication?

Notes:

43. Do I have to pay for my own Pentobarbital Sodium prescription drugs?

Notes:

44. Will Pentobarbital Sodium cause a mood change?

Notes:

45. Do you have Pentobarbital Sodium prescription drugs I can take throughout the day?

Notes:

46. Should I take my Pentobarbital Sodium medications at a regular time each day?

Notes:

47. Do I need to take Pentobarbital Sodium medications?

Notes:

48. Have you heard any stories about buying Pentobarbital Sodium prescription drugs over the internet?

Notes:

49. Is there an effective way to prevent and treat without Pentobarbital Sodium prescription drugs?

Notes:

50. Are related potential conditions avoidable, or do they require topical or other prescription medications?

Notes:

51. Can I take this Pentobarbital Sodium medicine if I am pregnant?

Notes:

52. What is the Prescription Drug Monitoring Database and who is using it?

Notes:

53. Can I take _____ with Pentobarbital Sodium prescription drugs?

Notes:

54. They say _____ not to take this with Pentobarbital Sodium prescription medication, but do you think it will hurt me?

Notes:

55. Who can assist with Pentobarbital Sodium medication reminders?

Notes:

56. Can my child have his or her Pentobarbital Sodium medication administered during the school day?

Notes:

57. Who should NOT take Pentobarbital Sodium medication?

Notes:

58. Do pill boxes help prevent Pentobarbital Sodium medication errors?

Notes:

59. Are all Pentobarbital Sodium prescription drugs covered under health care plans?

Notes:

60. Should I bring a list of medications and allergies?

Notes:

61. Are there any counter-indications about taking this supplement while taking any prescription drugs?

Notes:

62. So who approves these Pentobarbital Sodium medications?

Notes:

63. Who gets Pentobarbital Sodium, and when?

Notes:

64. Is Pentobarbital Sodium the right medication?

Notes:

65. Are you aware of my personal medical history including current medications, allergies, and other considerations or limitations?

Notes:

66. What is this Pentobarbital Sodium medication for, why am I taking it?

Notes:

67. Are there any risks or side effects?

Notes:

68. Do you know of any medications available out there that would help me be more comfortable?

Notes:

69. What should you do if I've messed up with my Pentobarbital Sodium medication?

Notes:

70. Who is accountable for my Pentobarbital Sodium prescription drug use?

Notes:

71. Do I HAVE to be on Pentobarbital Sodium medication?

Notes:

72. Is switching from one biologic medication to another effective?

Notes:

73. Which one of Pentobarbital Sodium medications is better for me than the others?

Notes:

74. Will taking Pentobarbital Sodium medication effect my mission call?

Notes:

75. May an employer ask all employees what prescription medications they are taking?

Notes:

76. Are there less intrusive, harmless and effective solutions instead of Pentobarbital Sodium prescription drugs?

Notes:

77. Should I expect a dependance on a medication which provides relief?

Notes:

78. Will I have to take my medications forever?

Notes:

79. Who is eligible to receive Pentobarbital Sodium prescription drug help?

Notes:

80. Do we have to do this test now?

Notes:

81. Should I eat while taking specialized Pentobarbital Sodium prescription drugs?

Notes:

82. Who is at risk for Pentobarbital Sodium prescription drug addiction?

Notes:

83. Who can get Medicare Pentobarbital Sodium prescription drug coverage?

Notes:

84. Are nutritional supplements safe to take if I am taking Pentobarbital Sodium prescription medications?

Notes:

85. What kinds of medications will I need to take and what if they don't work?

Notes:

86. Will my Pentobarbital Sodium prescription drugs build up toxins in my body?

Notes:

87. Are Pentobarbital Sodium medications effective?

Notes:

88. Is _____ a side effect of Pentobarbital Sodium medication and is it permanent?

Notes:

CHAPTER #2: WHAT:

INTENT: What do I need to know about Pentobarbital Sodium (What will it do for me and what can I expect.)

1. What if Pentobarbital Sodium medication makes me gain weight?

Notes:

2. What's the best mix for me of home remedies, over the counter (OTC) drugs and ointments and Pentobarbital Sodium prescription drugs?

Notes:

3. What is Pentobarbital Sodium medication for?

Notes:

4. What should I do if I experience side effects from the Pentobarbital Sodium?

Notes:

5. What is the best approach if I forget to take this Pentobarbital Sodium medication?

Notes:

6. What is the proper course of treatment for me?

Notes:

7. What about my current medications or allergies and the effect on it of Pentobarbital Sodium?

Notes:

8. What should I do if I have other prescription drug coverage and want to join Medicare First?

Notes:

9. What are my risks of accidentally taking an overdose of Pentobarbital Sodium prescription drugs?

Notes:

10. What else could I be doing to stay healthy and prevent disease?

Notes:

11. What if I am unhappy with the results of Pentobarbital Sodium medication?

Notes:

12. What is the brand name for the drug Pentobarbital Sodium?

Notes:

13. What are my Pentobarbital Sodium medication options?

Notes:

14. How will you know what medications I am on?

Notes:

15. What medications on the market, OTC or Pentobarbital Sodium prescription, can become harmful over time and would be dangerous if used well past the expiration date?

Notes:

16. What does my Pentobarbital Sodium medication look like?

Notes:

17. In what way can mindfulness or meditation be useful?

Notes:

18. What is the way to get my life back on track, without the unwanted side effects of Pentobarbital Sodium prescription drugs?

Notes:

19. What happens if I stop using Pentobarbital Sodium cold-turkey?

Notes:

20. Apart from Pentobarbital Sodium medication, what are other components of your management plan?

Notes:

21. What does a Pentobarbital Sodium medication error involve?

Notes:

22. What could be a natural alternative to more over-the-counter and Pentobarbital Sodium prescription drugs?

Notes:

23. Is Pentobarbital Sodium safe when breastfeeding, what are the effects on nursing?

Notes:

24. What are the different treatment options?

Notes:

25. What are other treatment options?

Notes:

26. What really works as well as these Pentobarbital Sodium medications, are there alternatives?

Notes:

27. What exactly leads one to get dependent on Pentobarbital Sodium prescription drugs?

Notes:

28. What is the name of my Pentobarbital Sodium medication?

Notes:

29. What are the adverse health effects from Pentobarbital Sodium prescription drugs?

Notes:

30. What causes my condition?

Notes:

31. At what point would you recommend Pentobarbital Sodium prescription drugs, alternative therapies, or surgery?

Notes:

32. What is the name of my condition, are there any other names it's known by?

Notes:

33. What's the difference between all of the Pentobarbital Sodium's class medications?

Notes:

34. What is the safest way to dispose of unwanted medications?

Notes:

35. What kind of Pentobarbital Sodium medications do the varying plans offer and how much can I save?

Notes:

36. Do I need to change what I eat or stop any Pentobarbital Sodium medications before doing a test?

Notes:

37. What is the effect of Pentobarbital Sodium on drowsiness?

Notes:

38. What will a negative result mean?

Notes:

39. What do I need to know about making the most of this Pentobarbital Sodium prescription?

Notes:

40. What Pentobarbital Sodium prescription drugs have serious side effects?

Notes:

41. What sort of Pentobarbital Sodium prescription drug benefit is included?

Notes:

42. What is the prescription drug of choice for breakthrough pain meds?

Notes:

43. What kind of resources do I have available to me?

Notes:

44. What Pentobarbital Sodium medication should I take?

Notes:

45. What types of vitamins and supplements should I be taking?

Notes:

46. What are the important warnings for males taking Pentobarbital Sodium?

Notes:

47. What if I have tried various home remedies, over-the-counter medications or even Pentobarbital Sodium prescription medications with no help?

Notes:

48. What Pentobarbital Sodium medications are used?

Notes:

49. What are the side effects of the Pentobarbital Sodium medication?

Notes:

50. What if Pentobarbital Sodium medication has changed since the application form was sent in?

Notes:

51. Is treatment required, if so - what is it?

Notes:

52. What prescription drugs are you yourself taking?

Notes:

53. What will happen if I don't have the treatment?

Notes:

54. What about Pentobarbital Sodium prescription drug coverage?

Notes:

55. What lifestyle changes can change my condition?

Notes:

56. What are some of the best non prescription medications I can give a try?

Notes:

57. What is my Pentobarbital Sodium prescription drug benefit?

Notes:

58. What's the probability that my Pentobarbital Sodium medication is causing my symptoms?

Notes:

59. What are the important warnings for females taking Pentobarbital Sodium?

Notes:

60. What are the Pentobarbital Sodium medications I can take?

Notes:

61. What kind of expectations should I have?

Notes:

62. What medications should I ask for?

Notes:

63. How will I benefit from working out in relation to my use of Pentobarbital Sodium prescription medication, and what type of exercise would you recommend?

Notes:

64. What else can I do to treat my condition?

Notes:

65. What medications can Pentobarbital Sodium interact with?

Notes:

66. What is a generic Pentobarbital Sodium medication?

Notes:

67. What medications are available to treat my condition?

Notes:

68. What will a positive result mean?

Notes:

69. What's to lose by trying another Pentobarbital Sodium class medication?

Notes:

70. In what situation would I need to go for counseling if I'm receiving medication treatment?

Notes:

71. What can I expect from Pentobarbital Sodium medication?

Notes:

72. Will I need medication and what will it be, Pentobarbital Sodium and/or anything else?

Notes:

73. What if I am taking vitamins or over-the-counter drugs that could affect my Pentobarbital Sodium prescription drugs?

Notes:

74. What Pentobarbital Sodium's class medication can I take best?

Notes:

75. What kind of experience with these issues do you have?

Notes:

76. What's your go-to question for your own doctor?

Notes:

77. What happens with my prescriptions for Pentobarbital Sodium medications while I am travelling overseas, how to get and fulfil those?

Notes:

78. What are the side effects?

Notes:

79. What happens if I have to cut my Pentobarbital Sodium pills in half to make them last longer or skip a day of medication because I can't afford to buy it as often as it's prescribed?

Notes:

80. What is a 25/50 percent Pentobarbital Sodium prescription drug plan?

Notes:

81. What medications have you yourself used in the past to make yourself better?

Notes:

82. What if I take Pentobarbital Sodium prescription drugs and get little or no relief?

Notes:

83. What should you, as my doctor, know before prescribing Pentobarbital Sodium medication?

Notes:

84. What sexual response side effects can I expect from these Pentobarbital Sodium medications?

Notes:

85. What side effects can Pentobarbital Sodium medication cause?

Notes:

86. What will my Pentobarbital Sodium medication do for me?

Notes:

87. What about Pentobarbital Sodium's interactions with my medications?

Notes:

88. What about side effects of Pentobarbital Sodium?

Notes:

89. What can I do to prevent my condition from recurring or worsening?

Notes:

90. What do you recommend to do with Pentobarbital Sodium medication adherence being difficult for me since my busy life pulls me in multiple directions - can you help me understand the ramifications of non-adherence?

Notes:

91. What is a prescription drug error and how often and why do these errors occur??

Notes:

92. What are good reasons to not take my Pentobarbital Sodium prescription medication?

Notes:

93. What is the evidence for this treatment?

Notes:

94. What is are food or drinks you recommend not to be taken with Pentobarbital Sodium prescription medications?

Notes:

95. What is the branded prescription drug fee?

Notes:

96. What will happen to me without Pentobarbital

Sodium prescription drugs, diet, exercise, or nutritional supplements?

Notes:

97. Can you help me understand how much of my Pentobarbital Sodium prescription drugs, equipment and services will be covered by my insurance and what I will have to pay?

Notes:

98. What if I am currently taking some other prescription medications?

Notes:

99. What other prescription drugs should I avoid while taking my Pentobarbital Sodium medicines?

Notes:

100. What are my options if I have difficulty paying for Pentobarbital Sodium prescription drugs?

Notes:

101. What are my options in relation to Pentobarbital Sodium medication, surgical procedures or remedy?

Notes:

102. For what reasons would I have to be off Pentobarbital Sodium medication and for how long?

Notes:

103. What is the test for?

Notes:

104. What if I'm taking other medication?

Notes:

105. What to eat, or what to use as a medication together with Pentobarbital Sodium?

Notes:

106. What will this test tell us?

Notes:

107. What prescription medications or off the shelf medicinal products would cause ringing in the ears?

Notes:

108. What questions haven't I asked that I should have?

Notes:

109. What are the benefits of having the test?

Notes:

110. What about my regular medications, any interference with Pentobarbital Sodium?

Notes:

111. What is my outcome?

Notes:

112. What are the causes of Pentobarbital Sodium prescription drug abuse?

Notes:

113. What are your thoughts on hypnotherapy and Pentobarbital Sodium?

Notes:

114. What sources can I trust?

Notes:

115. What should I know about Pentobarbital Sodium medication?

Notes:

116. What are the signs and symptoms related to Pentobarbital Sodium addiction?

Notes:

117. How do I book in to have the test and what is the usual waiting period?

Notes:

118. What is the easiest way to obtain the latest information about Pentobarbital Sodium prescription drugs?

Notes:

119. What about taking a new Pentobarbital Sodium medication?

Notes:

120. What replacement medications can you suggest for Pentobarbital Sodium?

Notes:

121. What happens if I don't do anything?

Notes:

122. What if I have been taking Pentobarbital Sodium

medication with little to no relief?

Notes:

123. Besides Pentobarbital Sodium medication, what else to do?

Notes:

124. What if my prescription Pentobarbital Sodium medication is lost or stolen?

Notes:

125. What kind of medication will I have to take, Pentobarbital Sodium or anything else?

Notes:

126. What if I have an allergic reaction to Pentobarbital Sodium?

Notes:

127. What's next?

Notes:

128. What other sources are available, who can I talk to about this?

Notes:

129. What would you do if you were me?

Notes:

130. What are the Pentobarbital Sodium medication side-effects?

Notes:

131. What should I do if I miss my regular dose of Pentobarbital Sodium?

Notes:

132. How do scientists determine whether the chemical compounds in Pentobarbital Sodium prescription medications do what they're claimed to do?

Notes:

133. I want to read more about my condition. What online sources should I trust?

Notes:

134. What types of Pentobarbital Sodium medications are available?

Notes:

135. What are your experiences with Pentobarbital Sodium prescription drugs?

Notes:

136. What other Pentobarbital Sodium-like medications are in this class?

Notes:

137. What non-Pentobarbital Sodium medications or vitamins should I take to speed up my healing?

Notes:

138. What are the dosages of the Pentobarbital Sodium medication?

Notes:

139. What is the effect of Pentobarbital Sodium on infertility?

Notes:

140. What is a generic Pentobarbital Sodium medication or drug, what does that term mean and what can it do for me?

Notes:

141. What does this sign on my Pentobarbital Sodium prescription drug imply?

Notes:

142. What other drugs could interact with Pentobarbital Sodium medication?

Notes:

143. Is it possible that my employer may look at what Pentobarbital Sodium prescription medications I'm taking?

Notes:

144. What should I expect after a procedure in terms of soreness, what to watch for, Pentobarbital Sodium medication, bathing, and level of activity?

Notes:

145. What is the safest way to dispose of unused prescription Pentobarbital Sodium medication?

Notes:

146. What is Pentobarbital Sodium prescription drug detox?

Notes:

147. What if I'm already on medication and have side-effects from the Pentobarbital Sodium?

Notes:

148. What would happen if I don't take the Pentobarbital Sodium, would my health get worse?

Notes:

149. What if the Pentobarbital Sodium medications produce unwelcome or harmful effects?

Notes:

150. What outcome should I expect?

Notes:

151. What will be the net effect of Pentobarbital Sodium medications for me?

Notes:

152. What can I do to remember to take my Pentobarbital Sodium medication?

Notes:

153. What can I do to help win the war on prescription drug abuse?

Notes:

154. What can parents and other adults do to help prevent prescription drug abuse among youth?

Notes:

155. What is the nature of the Pentobarbital Sodium medications prescribed?

Notes:

156. What about alcohol and its effect on Pentobarbital Sodium prescription drugs?

Notes:

157. What Pentobarbital Sodium-like medications are safe to take during pregnancy?

Notes:

CHAPTER #3: WHERE:

INTENT: Where to next (Where can I find more information. Do i need a second opionion. What happens with tests.)

1. Does Pentobarbital Sodium medication work?

Notes:

2. What if I refuse the prescribed Pentobarbital Sodium medication?

Notes:

3. Are you considering a trial of Pentobarbital Sodium medications and/or anything else?

Notes:

4. Where can I get my Pentobarbital Sodium prescription medications filled?

Notes:

5. Is this worth getting Pentobarbital Sodium medication for?

Notes:

6. Is there anything I can do to improve it myself?

Notes:

7. Where are others buying their Pentobarbital Sodium prescription medications?

Notes:

8. What if my current Pentobarbital Sodium prescription drugs are not on the formulary or are limited on the formulary?

Notes:

9. Can we really know what is in Pentobarbital Sodium prescription drugs?

Notes:

10. Are my prescription drugs also available in a generic version?

Notes:

11. Is there a better way to easily adhere to Pentobarbital Sodium prescription medication regimens?

Notes:

12. Are there any risks involved in having this test?

Notes:

13. Do some Pentobarbital Sodium prescription drugs cost more or have additional requirements for coverage?

Notes:

14. Can I take Pentobarbital Sodium medication?

Notes:

15. Do I need to see any other health professionals - such as specialists - physiotherapists - dieticians or dentists?

Notes:

16. Will you try and keep my Pentobarbital Sodium medications at a level where I can function?

Notes:

17. Can alternative medicine counter Pentobarbital Sodium prescription medication and over-the-counters with their limited effectiveness and potential side effects?

Notes:

18. Should I take Pentobarbital Sodium with other medications?

Notes:

19. What can I expect about the absorption of active ingredients in my Pentobarbital Sodium prescription medications?

Notes:

20. How does a Pentobarbital Sodium medication reminder service work?

Notes:

21. Can I travel to _____ with prescription drugs used as medication for my condition?

Notes:

22. How do I avoid getting in a place where I need so many prescription drugs to function?

Notes:

23. Can my condition come back?

Notes:

24. Which medication for my condition is right for me?

Notes:

25. Where do I go if I've run out of money and desperately need Pentobarbital Sodium medication or a medical procedure?

Notes:

26. Are herbal supplements safe when I am taking other Pentobarbital Sodium prescription medications?

Notes:

27. Is there a non-prescription Pentobarbital Sodium medication you might recommend?

Notes:

28. Where can I find info about taking more than one prescription medications together with Pentobarbital Sodium?

Notes:

29. When you prescribe Pentobarbital Sodium prescription medication for my condition, how do you weigh the side effects?

Notes:

30. Could thePentobarbital Sodium prescription drug I am taking now be the cause of a few extra pounds?

Notes:

31. Is there an alternative medication?

Notes:

32. What are the differences between generic and brand medications?

Notes:

33. Do I really need this test?

Notes:

34. Is it normal to feel this way?

Notes:

35. What if I am out of the country and lose my Pentobarbital Sodium prescription medications?

Notes:

36. Will any of the current Pentobarbital Sodium medications I am taking increase my risk for _____?

Notes:

37. Who monitors the safety and effectiveness of Pentobarbital Sodium prescription drugs?

Notes:

38. Are all drug-drug interactions limited to Pentobarbital Sodium prescription medications?

Notes:

39. What does 50 deductible for brand name

prescription drugs mean?

Notes:

40. Please explain, what are the differences between generic and brand Pentobarbital Sodium medications?

Notes:

41. Should I lock up my Pentobarbital Sodium prescription drugs?

Notes:

42. Where can I buy Pentobarbital Sodium prescription drugs cheaper?

Notes:

43. Which Pentobarbital Sodium medications are addictive?

Notes:

44. How can you help me when I suffer from

chronic pain, but am leery about taking prescription medication to help it?

Notes:

45. Is there a certain Pentobarbital Sodium or other medication that can improve my symptoms?

Notes:

46. What f I have any allergies to food, medications or things in the environment?

Notes:

47. What are the best ways that do not require prescription medications to fall asleep faster?

Notes:

48. Do you have my vital records and medications up to date?

Notes:

49. Precisely what are some good reasons

Pentobarbital Sodium prescription drugs can be recommended?

Notes:

50. Are the brands of Pentobarbital Sodium prescription drugs I take covered?

Notes:

51. How do prescription medications compare to herbal forms of treatment for my condition?

Notes:

52. Will I be on Pentobarbital Sodium medication forever?

Notes:

53. Have you instructed patients to discontinue taking their Pentobarbital Sodium, or other prescription drugs?

Notes:

54. Could you write it down?

Notes:

55. Is this normal or should I see a shrink for Pentobarbital Sodium medication?

Notes:

56. How to take Pentobarbital Sodium medication?

Notes:

57. Where would I store my Pentobarbital Sodium medications?

Notes:

58. If remedies help, what is the nature of Pentobarbital Sodium medications and where could one go to explore them?

Notes:

59. I am paid to _____ for a living, will my performance improve or decrease while using

Pentobarbital Sodium prescription drugs?

Notes:

60. Are there generic equivalents available for my Pentobarbital Sodium prescription drugs?

Notes:

61. Do Pentobarbital Sodium medications accelerate aging?

Notes:

62. Can I schedule my surgery for the morning?

Notes:

63. Will grapefruit affect my Pentobarbital Sodium medications?

Notes:

64. Will any of the supplements that have been prescribed for me interfere with any Pentobarbital Sodium prescription medications I may already be on?

Notes:

65. Can I take _____ with Pentobarbital Sodium prescription drugs?

Notes:

66. Could any of the Pentobarbital Sodium medications contribute to impotence?

Notes:

67. If I take Pentobarbital Sodium prescription drugs long term, do I run the risk of becoming addicted?

Notes:

68. Is it probable to uncover how to deal with _____ without taking prescription medication?

Notes:

69. Can my Pentobarbital Sodium medication be delivered if I don't attend appointments?

Notes:

70. Can I still take my current medications?

Notes:

71. Can I drink alcohol while I am taking Pentobarbital Sodium?

Notes:

72. Should I rely on Pentobarbital Sodium, natural cures or over the counter medication?

Notes:

73. Will Pentobarbital Sodium medication be the proper strength?

Notes:

74. Will Pentobarbital Sodium prescriptions drugs affect urine drug screen?

Notes:

75. Where should I get my Pentobarbital Sodium prescription drugs?

Notes:

76. Where would you send your partner or children?

Notes:

77. Does my policy cover Pentobarbital Sodium prescription drugs?

Notes:

78. Can a Pentobarbital Sodium prescription drug card preserve me cash?

Notes:

79. Will Pentobarbital Sodium interfere with other prescription medications?

Notes:

80. Which Pentobarbital Sodium-related prescription drugs are most dangerous?

Notes:

81. Will Pentobarbital Sodium medication control my symptoms adequately?

Notes:

82. Can all doctors prescribe Pentobarbital Sodium Prescription Medication?

Notes:

83. I am on prescription Pentobarbital Sodium medication, can I still detox?

Notes:

84. If I get concerned with the high cost of medical care and Pentobarbital Sodium prescriptions drugs, will you help me explore my options for a more natural approach like seeking help from acupuncturists, naturopaths, chiropractors?

Notes:

85. Where can I get more info about that?

Notes:

86. What are generic alternatives for my Pentobarbital Sodium prescription drugs?

Notes:

87. Where can US citizens buy their prescription drugs online from legally, in confidence, and under which conditions?

Notes:

88. Do Pentobarbital Sodium prescription drugs create new mental problems?

Notes:

CHAPTER #4: WHEN:

INTENT: When should I take or stop taking Pentobarbital Sodium and how (When should I take it, stop taking it and how.)

1. When can seniors join a Pentobarbital Sodium prescription drug plan?

Notes:

2. When I have been on the same amount of Pentobarbital Sodium medication for years – when should that be re-evaluated?

Notes:

3. Is it true that an online pharmacy can save me money on Pentobarbital Sodium prescription drugs?

Notes:

4. Can Pentobarbital Sodium medications or my health problems keep me awake?

Notes:

5. Are my Pentobarbital Sodium medications safe to use while breastfeeding?

Notes:

6. Can I take Pentobarbital Sodium with other medications?

Notes:

7. Is it possible to lower my blood pressure without taking prescription drugs?

Notes:

8. How and when should I take my Pentobarbital Sodium medication?

Notes:

9. Do you earn bonuses based on performance?

Notes:

10. Are there other ways to treat my condition?

Notes:

11. What does one do when the only real help, the only Pentobarbital Sodium medication available, no longer works?

Notes:

12. How do I deal with any Pentobarbital Sodium prescription medication when a side effect may be stated as 'may cause nausea or vomiting'?

Notes:

13. I take daily prescription medications, may I take my pills before I have my blood drawn?

Notes:

14. When could Pentobarbital Sodium medication not be working anymore?

Notes:

15. Can Reiki be used when taking Pentobarbital Sodium medications?

Notes:

16. What medications do I need to stop and when?

Notes:

17. Should I have a current emergency contact form and a list of health conditions and medications readily available?

Notes:

18. When should I be on Pentobarbital Sodium medication?

Notes:

19. Does it matter at what time I use my Pentobarbital Sodium medication?

Notes:

20. Is Pentobarbital Sodium a medicine with real evidence?

Notes:

21. Do I really need to take this Pentobarbital Sodium medication?

Notes:

22. Do generic medications have the exact same ingredients?

Notes:

23. How do I use my insurance to get discounts on my Pentobarbital Sodium prescription medication?

Notes:

24. Is it either / or when it comes to natural medicines and Pentobarbital Sodium prescription drugs?

Notes:

25. Are there any known Pentobarbital Sodium prescription medication and chia seeds side effects when they are combined?

Notes:

26. Are extended-release (ER) opioid medications optimum pain medications?

Notes:

27. When might herbal and nutritional therapies be a good alternative to over-the-counter and Pentobarbital Sodium prescription medications for people with my condition?

Notes:

28. Will Pentobarbital Sodium prescription medications cause weight loss?

Notes:

29. Where I can get a Pentobarbital Sodium prescription drug?

Notes:

30. Is Pentobarbital Sodium medication the only answer for me?

Notes:

31. If I need a surgery and I did go ahead with the surgery, how might that affect the Pentobarbital Sodium medications I take?

Notes:

32. Are there medications available that really fix the underlying cause of my condition?

Notes:

33. When should I stop taking Pentobarbital Sodium medication?

Notes:

34. Do I need to prepare for the test (for example - by fasting beforehand)?

Notes:

35. When should I take this Pentobarbital Sodium medicine?

Notes:

36. Would increasing the dose of Pentobarbital Sodium have a positive effect or would I be better off asking you to try some new medications?

Notes:

37. Can Pentobarbital Sodium prescription drugs cause problems during pregnancy?

Notes:

38. What are the active ingredients in Pentobarbital Sodium prescription medication?

Notes:

39. When is it appropriate and safe to prescribe Pentobarbital Sodium medication for my condition?

Notes:

40. When will I know that I am taking excessive pain medication?

Notes:

41. How long am I expected to take this Pentobarbital Sodium medication?

Notes:

42. When should I stop using Pentobarbital Sodium medication because of....?

Notes:

43. When did you graduate from medical school?

Notes:

44. Is this necessary now?

Notes:

45. What is the safest prescription drug disposal method?

Notes:

46. How can I get Pentobarbital Sodium prescription drug coverage?

Notes:

47. Will St. John's Wort interfere with Pentobarbital Sodium prescription medications?

Notes:

48. Which of my medications cause the most weight gain?

Notes:

49. Are there any drug interactions if Pentobarbital Sodium is taken in combination with other

medications?

Notes:

50. Can the Pentobarbital Sodium medication cause substance abuse?

Notes:

51. Can I take ayurvedic products with Pentobarbital Sodium prescription medications?

Notes:

52. Are medication reminders only for prescription medications?

Notes:

53. Are Pentobarbital Sodium medications safe for young kids?

Notes:

54. Do individual policies pay for prescription Pentobarbital Sodium medications?

Notes:

55. What are the effects of Pentobarbital Sodium medications on cognition?

Notes:

56. If you have a Pentobarbital Sodium prescription drug in your pocket, outside of the container when arrested is that considered DUI?

Notes:

57. Should I really use this Pentobarbital Sodium medication?

Notes:

58. Where can I obtain a list of Pentobarbital Sodium prescription drugs that require prior approval?

Notes:

59. When and how will I get the results?

Notes:

60. Will it help when I tell you about all my current medications and vitamin and herbal supplements?

Notes:

61. Do I need this particular Pentobarbital Sodium medication?

Notes:

62. Is Pentobarbital Sodium as effective as other prescription medications?

Notes:

63. Can I take Pentobarbital Sodium with my other medications?

Notes:

64. Will you try and reach the primary reason for my problem before prescribing Pentobarbital Sodium medications to solve my particular signs and symptoms?

Notes:

65. Where are Pentobarbital Sodium prescription drug users getting their prescription filled locally?

Notes:

66. Will Pentobarbital Sodium interact with any other medicines I take - including any vitamins - herbal medicine or other complementary medicine?

Notes:

67. Can anyone get these Pentobarbital Sodium prescription drugs?

Notes:

68. What happens if I am willing to try new medications if the current Pentobarbital Sodium ones are not working?

Notes:

69. Will my Pentobarbital Sodium prescription drug

have a drivers warning on it?

Notes:

70. Can using too much or too little Pentobarbital Sodium prescription drugs harm my health?

Notes:

71. Will I be able to do _____ after treatment?

Notes:

72. When does Pentobarbital Sodium medication begin working?

Notes:

73. I am feeling anxious and/or blue lately. Is this normal, can you help me?

Notes:

74. Will I be able to carry enough prescription medications to avoid any health emergencies?

Notes:

75. Is it likely to get worse, or is it likely to get better?

Notes:

76. What medications are safe for me to take during my pregnancy?

Notes:

77. Do I really need this treatment?

Notes:

78. Do Pentobarbital Sodium medications work for everybody?

Notes:

79. What are some great ways to help remind me when to take Pentobarbital Sodium medications?

Notes:

80. Will any supplements interact with my Pentobarbital Sodium prescription drugs?

Notes:

81. Is it legal to buy Pentobarbital Sodium prescription medications online?

Notes:

82. Are there any alternative tests?

Notes:

83. How/when do I get test results?

Notes:

84. Will you keep my current medications the same?

Notes:

85. When does this Pentobarbital Sodium medication

expire?

Notes:

86. Should I stop my Pentobarbital Sodium medications before any procedure?

Notes:

87. Are Pentobarbital Sodium prescription medications included in my monthly insurance fee?

Notes:

CHAPTER #5: WHY:

INTENT: Why do I need Pentobarbital Sodium (Are there Alternatives. Why do I need it. Which symptoms does it medicate.)

1. What if my religion condones the use of Pentobarbital Sodium medications?

Notes:

2. Who typically, signed up for the Medicare Prescription Drug plan, are already hitting the gap in coverage known as the doughnut hole - and what is my risk of hitting the doughnut hole?

Notes:

3. Should I stop taking my Pentobarbital Sodium medication(s) before a evaluation or a surgery?

Notes:

4. Are any nutrients depleted by this Pentobarbital Sodium medication?

Notes:

5. Which Pentobarbital Sodium prescription drugs can be addictive?

Notes:

6. Why are you doing this test?

Notes:

7. Why are we doing these tests?

Notes:

8. I feel like I need more medication, will you as my doctor be able to support me with my requests?

Notes:

9. How will the treatment effect the medications that I currently take for _____?

Notes:

10. Am I up to date on my routine health maintenance?

Notes:

11. Why can't I buy some prescription drugs online?

Notes:

12. Is this something I should worry about or is it just a side effect of Pentobarbital Sodium?

Notes:

13. Will I need any Pentobarbital Sodium medication after surgery?

Notes:

14. How does my child at an out-of-state school obtain prescription drugs?

Notes:

15. Can I take Pentobarbital Sodium with prescription medication or with an underlying medical condition?

Notes:

16. Why is Pentobarbital Sodium medication prescribed?

Notes:

17. Does the Pentobarbital Sodium medicine need to be stored in the fridge?

Notes:

18. May I bring multiple prescription medications to take while I am in custody?

Notes:

19. Why are Pentobarbital Sodium medications so popular?

Notes:

20. Are there any side effects from taking nutritional supplements and Pentobarbital Sodium prescription medications at the same time?

Notes:

21. Could I have afforded it without Pentobarbital Sodium prescription drug insurance?

Notes:

22. Why would I need Pentobarbital Sodium prescription medication reminders?

Notes:

23. What if I start depending on antidepressants, alcohol, or other medications to calm me down or help me sleep?

Notes:

24. Do you know all of the risks Pentobarbital Sodium prescription drugs might pose?

Notes:

25. Why and when use acupuncture for treating pain instead of, or combined with, taking pain medication?

Notes:

26. Will kinesiology interfere with Pentobarbital Sodium medication?

Notes:

27. Can enzymes be taken with other Pentobarbital Sodium prescription medications?

Notes:

28. How do I get my Pentobarbital Sodium medication without prescription drug coverage?

Notes:

29. Should I be concerned about all the Pentobarbital Sodium medication I need to take to stay on top of my health problems?

Notes:

30. Can you help me save money on my Pentobarbital Sodium prescription medication?

Notes:

31. Why does a prescription drug require authorization by a qualified professional and others do not?

Notes:

32. What is the effect of my Pentobarbital Sodium use if I smoke?

Notes:

33. Will Pentobarbital Sodium prescription medications cause gum problems?

Notes:

34. What do you turn to for adjunctive medications, usually?

Notes:

35. Why are you giving me a blood test - and what will the results tell us?

Notes:

36. Should I get a second opinion?

Notes:

37. Why have my bowel habits/appetite/mood/sex drive/etc changed?

Notes:

38. Does my condition have to be treated with Pentobarbital Sodium prescription drugs?

Notes:

39. When is it time to think about why I'm on these Pentobarbital Sodium drugs?

Notes:

40. Why is this Pentobarbital Sodium medication prescribed?

Notes:

41. Why go the Pentobarbital Sodium medication route?

Notes:

42. Is Pentobarbital Sodium a slow releasing medication?

Notes:

43. If I am stranded abroad and run out of my normal Pentobarbital Sodium prescription medication, am I covered for this?

Notes:

44. Is there an effective herbal alternative or supplement to Pentobarbital Sodium medication?

Notes:

45. Will I require any Pentobarbital Sodium prescription drugs?

Notes:

46. Could Pentobarbital Sodium prescription medications cause a false positive on a test?

Notes:

47. Are there any other restrictions on Pentobarbital Sodium prescription drug coverage?

Notes:

48. Can or should I take my Pentobarbital Sodium medications at breakfast with my grapefruit juice?

Notes:

49. Do we have to do this now - or can we revisit it

later?

Notes:

50. Will Pentobarbital Sodium meet my expectations?

Notes:

51. How do you handle potential prescription drug addiction and flow-on depression?

Notes:

52. Why is Pentobarbital Sodium a prescription drug?

Notes:

53. Will taking Pentobarbital Sodium make me irritable?

Notes:

54. Are there safe Pentobarbital Sodium-class prescription drugs available?

Notes:

55. Can I take the generic version of your prescription drugs?

Notes:

56. Why does my family's medical history matter, and what should I do about it?

Notes:

57. Is self-administration of Pentobarbital Sodium medication allowed?

Notes:

58. What exactly is this Pentobarbital Sodium medication for in my case and how do you think it is working so well?

Notes:

59. Will these Pentobarbital Sodium medications cause weight gain?

Notes:

60. Is Pentobarbital Sodium compatible with my current prescribed medication?

Notes:

61. Will I get possible side neuritis of Pentobarbital Sodium medications?

Notes:

62. Can you suggest alternatives to Pentobarbital Sodium prescription medication?

Notes:

63. Can enzymes be taken when a person is on Pentobarbital Sodium prescription medications?

Notes:

64. Do you think that I may have or get a problem with Pentobarbital Sodium medications?

Notes:

65. Why do I need Pentobarbital Sodium medicine?

Notes:

66. Should I be worried about this lump/spot/_____?

Notes:

67. If I take a Pentobarbital Sodium medication, will it require more medication to counter the side effects?

Notes:

68. Are there any other precautions or warnings for this Pentobarbital Sodium medication?

Notes:

69. Is there anything else I should be asking?

Notes:

70. Can you inform me about nutrition, exercise, Pentobarbital Sodium medications and

complications?

Notes:

71. What if I am affected by anxiety and don't like the thought of taking prescription medications?

Notes:

72. Will Pentobarbital Sodium have an effect on nausea?

Notes:

73. How do Pentobarbital Sodium prescription drugs work?

Notes:

74. What is the difference between a natural herbal supplement and a prescription drug?

Notes:

75. Pentobarbital Sodium is most definitely a prescription drug?

Notes:

76. Is there financial help for Pentobarbital Sodium prescription drugs?

Notes:

77. Why is it important to take my Pentobarbital Sodium prescription medication exactly as prescribed?

Notes:

78. Is there a Pentobarbital Sodium prescription drug guide on the internet?

Notes:

79. Why would I, while regularly taking prescription medications, have to approach grapefruit consumption with caution?

Notes:

80. If I have been taking the same prescription

drugs for a long time, when is it time to evaluate?

Notes:

81. Can nutritional yeasts, especially brewers yeast, interact with Pentobarbital Sodium medications?

Notes:

82. If I use prescription drugs, can I be arrested for DUI?

Notes:

83. Why is buying Pentobarbital Sodium prescription drugs without a prescription dangerous?

Notes:

84. Where else can I go for Pentobarbital Sodium prescription medication, what are my options?

Notes:

85. Is it safe getting pregnant while on Pentobarbital Sodium medications?

Notes:

86. If I want to talk to a specialist in Pentobarbital Sodium prescription drugs, where do I go?

Notes:

87. Can I use this app I found?

Notes:

88. Why do I need to manage Pentobarbital Sodium medications?

Notes:

CHAPTER #6: HOW:

INTENT: How will Pentobarbital Sodium affect me (How will it affect me negatively. How do I know if its a problem for me.)

1. How can I dispose of my Pentobarbital Sodium prescription drugs safely?

Notes:

2. How can I support my bone health naturally with and without medication?

Notes:

3. How effective is this treatment?

Notes:

4. How's my weight?

Notes:

5. How long does the prescription drug Pentobarbital Sodium stay in your system?

Notes:

6. How is the Pentobarbital Sodium medication delivered?

Notes:

7. So how do you know if you, or someone you love is having problems with Pentobarbital Sodium prescription drug abuse?

Notes:

8. How soon do I need to have the test?

Notes:

9. How to go about it if I want to use a lower dosage of Pentobarbital Sodium?

Notes:

10. How will Pentobarbital Sodium affect my sleeping pattern?

Notes:

11. Do you know how long it will take me to get my Pentobarbital Sodium medication?

Notes:

12. How often do I need to have the test done?

Notes:

13. Do you have research you can share on Pentobarbital Sodium prescription drug prices?

Notes:

14. How long does a Pentobarbital Sodium medication remain active in your body?

Notes:

15. How serious is this condition?

Notes:

16. Are there support groups for people with this problem and how would I contact them?

Notes:

17. How wide-ranging is the Pentobarbital Sodium prescription drug coverage?

Notes:

18. How is Pentobarbital Sodium medication supposed to help me?

Notes:

19. How do different Pentobarbital Sodium-class prescription medications work differently?

Notes:

20. How are Pentobarbital Sodium prescription drugs abused?

Notes:

21. How can Pentobarbital Sodium medication be detected?

Notes:

22. How long is it likely to last?

Notes:

23. How should I use this Pentobarbital Sodium medication?

Notes:

24. How long should I take Pentobarbital Sodium medication?

Notes:

25. How does Pentobarbital Sodium prescription drug abuse start?

Notes:

26. How do generic medications compare in quality to brand name drugs?

Notes:

27. How many surgeries do you perform each year?

Notes:

28. How can I learn more about my symptoms or condition?

Notes:

29. How do I know if I have permanent hair loss due to medication?

Notes:

30. Can I take over-the-counter drugs or are prescription drugs more effective?

Notes:

31. How does Pentobarbital Sodium interact with other medications?

Notes:

32. How do you handle children on Pentobarbital Sodium medication?

Notes:

33. How do I manage my Pentobarbital Sodium medications?

Notes:

34. How long do I have to take Pentobarbital Sodium medication?

Notes:

35. How accurate are the results of the test?

Notes:

36. How is the test done?

Notes:

37. How can I reduce or stop some of my medications?

Notes:

38. How do I take this Pentobarbital Sodium medication?

Notes:

39. Are there drugs to lift my mood, and how can this be achieved without prescription medications?

Notes:

40. How can I make sure I am sufficiently stocked with the Pentobarbital Sodium prescription medications I need?

Notes:

41. How do we order or pick up Pentobarbital Sodium medications?

Notes:

42. How do I dispose of Pentobarbital Sodium prescription medications?

Notes:

43. Does my plan cover the Pentobarbital Sodium prescription drugs I need?

Notes:

44. How do I get better without Pentobarbital Sodium medication?

Notes:

45. How about a new Pentobarbital Sodium-like prescription drug?

Notes:

46. How will I get the test results?

Notes:

47. Can Pentobarbital Sodium medication cause hair loss?

Notes:

48. How will I know if my current Pentobarbital Sodium Prescription Drug coverage is as good as the new Medicare Pentobarbital Sodium Prescription Drug coverage?

Notes:

49. How can my mental state successfully improve using medication or therapy?

Notes:

50. How long will the effect of Pentobarbital Sodium medication last?

Notes:

51. How can I opt for the generic alternative Pentobarbital Sodium medication that gives me the exact same results?

Notes:

52. In case I need pain relief, how can I get access to medical cannabis?

Notes:

53. How to store Pentobarbital Sodium medication?

Notes:

54. How long does the Pentobarbital Sodium medication last?

Notes:

55. How many patients with my condition have you treated?

Notes:

56. How should I take this Pentobarbital Sodium medication?

Notes:

57. How do the police suspect impairment by Pentobarbital Sodium prescription medication?

Notes:

58. Is it probable to find out how to deal with my condition without taking Pentobarbital Sodium prescription drugs?

Notes:

59. How soon should I come back?

Notes:

60. How quickly do I have to start the treatment?

Notes:

61. How will Pentobarbital Sodium affect the other medications that I'm taking?

Notes:

62. How should I take my Pentobarbital Sodium medication?

Notes:

63. How long do I need to take the Pentobarbital Sodium medicine for?

Notes:

64. My Pentobarbital Sodium medications, just how safe are they?

Notes:

65. How will I feel when I'm on Pentobarbital Sodium medications?

Notes:

66. How can Pentobarbital Sodium prescription drug abuse be recognized and stopped?

Notes:

67. How long will it take to get the results?

Notes:

68. So how do I save money on my Pentobarbital Sodium prescription drugs?

Notes:

69. What should I do if my symptoms are not relieved while taking Pentobarbital Sodium medication?

Notes:

70. How do I read the label on my Pentobarbital Sodium prescription drug package?

Notes:

71. How can I find a few methods that can help my condition without the use of Pentobarbital Sodium

prescription medication?

Notes:

72. Are my Pentobarbital Sodium prescription drugs FDA-approved?

Notes:

73. How should this Pentobarbital Sodium medication be taken?

Notes:

74. How should this Pentobarbital Sodium medication be stored?

Notes:

75. How will I hear about my test results?

Notes:

76. State prescription drug price web sites, how useful are they to me as a Pentobarbital Sodium consumer?

Notes:

77. How common is Pentobarbital Sodium prescription drug abuse?

Notes:

78. How long will I need the treatment for?

Notes:

79. How will I know if the Pentobarbital Sodium prescription and over-the-counter medications I take are interacting properly?

Notes:

80. How can I reduce my Pentobarbital Sodium prescription drug costs?

Notes:

81. How should I dispose of Pentobarbital Sodium prescription drugs?

Notes:

82. How do I manage multiple prescription medications together with Pentobarbital Sodium?

Notes:

83. Has anyone ever used this Pentobarbital Sodium medication?

Notes:

84. So I got a condition and a Pentobarbital Sodium medication – how am I, as a patient, supposed to manage treatment?

Notes:

85. Can this test diagnose a problem or will I need further testing?

Notes:

86. How does a person with dementia, living alone, manage her Pentobarbital Sodium medication?

Notes:

87. How often will I take the Pentobarbital Sodium medication?

Notes:

88. How often is the Pentobarbital Sodium medication taken?

Notes:

CHAPTER #7: HOW MUCH:

INTENT: How much will taking Pentobarbital Sodium cost me (In money and Pentobarbital Sodium's effect on quality of life.)

1. If I get sick - will you see me in the hospital?

Notes:

2. Um - can you explain that again?

Notes:

3. How much should I be charged for my Pentobarbital Sodium prescription medications?

Notes:

4. Because Medicare prescription drug coverage is so new to me, where can I get aid deciding on a program?

Notes:

5. Which prescription medications can cause impotence?

Notes:

6. Is it all right for me to take allergy medication?

Notes:

7. How do I get the Medicare Pentobarbital Sodium prescription drug benefit?

Notes:

8. How much can I use this Pentobarbital Sodium prescription drug plan?

Notes:

9. Can you slow down and keep it simple?

Notes:

10. How will I know when my Pentobarbital Sodium medications are working?

Notes:

11. Are generics available for all Pentobarbital Sodium prescription drugs?

Notes:

12. Is Pentobarbital Sodium a medication?

Notes:

13. Am I am worrying too much?

Notes:

14. How much do the Pentobarbital Sodium prescription drugs cost in this plan as compared to other plans?

Notes:

15. Do I take Pentobarbital Sodium prescription medications every day?

Notes:

16. Just how much do you know about the numerous types of Pentobarbital Sodium medications for the different types of my condition?

Notes:

17. Is Pentobarbital Sodium safe if taking medications for high blood pressure?

Notes:

18. Are Pentobarbital Sodium prescription drugs covered?

Notes:

19. Did you wash your hands?

Notes:

20. What herbs, supplements, foods, drinks or activities should I avoid while taking Pentobarbital Sodium medication?

Notes:

21. Which Pentobarbital Sodium's class related medication is the safest for me?

Notes:

22. Which part of Medicare will cover my Pentobarbital Sodium prescription drugs?

Notes:

23. Is Pentobarbital Sodium addictive?

Notes:

24. How much does it normally cost to get the surgery done, including all Pentobarbital Sodium medications and tests (ultrasounds,x-rays,medicines, hospital stay)?

Notes:

25. Is there an Over-The-Counter Medication that helps or maybe even can replace my Pentobarbital Sodium Prescription Medication?

Notes:

26. Should I join a Medicare Prescription Drug Plan even if I don't take many prescription drugs?

Notes:

27. How much will the plan cover for Pentobarbital Sodium prescription drugs?

Notes:

28. I'm taking prescription medication abroad, will this be covered if it is lost or I run out?

Notes:

29. Are non-prescription drugs less effective than Pentobarbital Sodium?

Notes:

30. How much is Medicare Pentobarbital Sodium prescription drug coverage worth?

Notes:

31. Are there any contraindications with Pentobarbital Sodium to other medications?

Notes:

32. What is a 3-Tier or 4-Tier prescription drug plan?

Notes:

33. So, is this a 'wow-factor' Pentobarbital Sodium medication?

Notes:

34. How much will this cost me?

Notes:

35. How much will the treatment cost?

Notes:

36. How much Pentobarbital Sodium prescription medication can I order from my pharmacy at one time?

Notes:

37. How much will my Pentobarbital Sodium prescription drugs cost me?

Notes:

38. Should I take Pentobarbital Sodium with food or drink?

Notes:

39. How much do I need to really understand about the interactions of my Pentobarbital Sodium prescription drugs?

Notes:

40. Will I feel doped from Pentobarbital Sodium?

Notes:

41. Does my plan have a Pentobarbital Sodium prescription drug formulary?

Notes:

42. How much does Pentobarbital Sodium cost?

Notes:

43. Would using Pentobarbital Sodium mean that I would need my other medications less?

Notes:

44. Common side effects of Pentobarbital Sodium include?

Notes:

45. Do I need a change in my Pentobarbital Sodium

medication?

Notes:

46. Do I need medication or surgery?

Notes:

47. Is there a Medicare Advantage plan provider who will cover my Pentobarbital Sodium prescription drug costs during the donut hole?

Notes:

48. Will the cost be covered by Medicare - my concession or Veterans Affairs card or by private health insurance?

Notes:

49. Is the Pentobarbital Sodium medication safe?

Notes:

50. May my employer ask me which Pentobarbital Sodium prescription medications I am taking?

Notes:

51. Do you know of any natural medication to help?

Notes:

52. Is this necessary right now?

Notes:

53. Can I ever be free of having to use prescription drugs?

Notes:

54. Can you explain my options for Medicare, Medicare/Medicaid, Disability, Supplemental Insurance, Part D Prescription Drug Plans, or Medicare Billings?

Notes:

55. Are Pentobarbital Sodium medications toxic?

Notes:

56. How much experience with this test or procedure do you have?

Notes:

57. Are there any side effects of taking Pentobarbital Sodium?

Notes:

58. Is sharing Pentobarbital Sodium prescription drugs illegal?

Notes:

59. How much will the test cost?

Notes:

60. How can I legally purchase Pentobarbital Sodium prescription medications from Canada?

Notes:

61. Where does my Pentobarbital Sodium prescription medication come from?

Notes:

62. Should I review my Medicare prescription drug plan choice every year?

Notes:

63. How much Pentobarbital Sodium medication can be brought through customs in case I travel?

Notes:

64. Can I share Pentobarbital Sodium prescription drugs?

Notes:

65. How much will it cost, will the cost be covered by the PBS - my concession or Veterans Affairs card or by private health insurance?

Notes:

66. Does switching Pentobarbital Sodium prescription drugs to over the counter as I age have any negative side effects?

Notes:

67. Will any tests be necessary while I am taking Pentobarbital Sodium medication?

Notes:

68. If acupuncture improves my condition, can I stop taking Pentobarbital Sodium prescription medications?

Notes:

69. What if I take pain medication for _____?

Notes:

70. Can I take Pentobarbital Sodium with my current medications?

Notes:

71. Would I need Pentobarbital Sodium prescription drugs that are not covered by insurance?

Notes:

72. Could natural products be just as effective as Pentobarbital Sodium prescription medications?

Notes:

73. How much am I likely to spend on Pentobarbital Sodium prescription drugs?

Notes:

74. Will I be able to take my prescription medications after surgery?

Notes:

75. Will Medicare be enough to cover the cost of my medical care, especially Pentobarbital Sodium prescription drugs?

Notes:

76. What would happen if I were suddenly unable to get access to my Pentobarbital Sodium prescription drugs?

Notes:

77. Are there any other medicines that can help me but without any side effects?

Notes:

78. What prescription drugs do I need covered?

Notes:

79. Do Pentobarbital Sodium medications deliver on their promise?

Notes:

80. How do I know how much my Pentobarbital Sodium prescription medication will be?

Notes:

81. Is it covered by Medicare - my concession or Veterans Affairs card or my private health insurance?

Notes:

82. Is it possible to start with a solution which is natural and effective and less expensive than Pentobarbital Sodium prescription medication?

Notes:

83. Can I continue to take Pentobarbital Sodium prescription drugs over 10, 20 and 30 years or more?

Notes:

84. Which Pentobarbital Sodium-like medication gives the most rapid relief?

Notes:

85. Regarding dosage, exactly how much of Pentobarbital Sodium can I take?

Notes:

86. How to get my Pentobarbital Sodium medication increased?

Notes:

87. Can Pentobarbital Sodium cause me to get a dry mouth as side effect?

Notes:

88. Do you offer treatment programs for those suffering from Pentobarbital Sodium prescription drug addiction?

Notes:

Index

148

limited 4, 59, 61, 65
listed   1
little   42, 50, 90
living   69, 128
locally 89
longer 41, 78
long-term   14
making   33
manage   111, 118, 128
management 15, 30
market 29
matter 80, 105
matters   1
mechanical   1
Medicaid   12, 140
medical   1, 4-5, 10-11, 20, 63, 74, 84, 97, 105, 122, 144
Medicare   10, 23, 27, 94, 121, 131, 134-136, 139-140, 142, 144, 146
medicate   94
medication   7-9, 12-13, 15, 18-22, 24, 26-31, 34-44, 46, 48-51, 53-55, 58-64, 67-69, 71-72, 74, 76-84, 86-88, 90, 92, 94-100, 102-103, 105-107, 109-110, 112-126, 128-129, 131-132, 134-137, 139-140, 142-143, 145-147
medicinal   47
medicine   5, 11, 17, 61, 80, 83, 89, 97, 107, 124
medicines   45, 81, 89, 134, 145
meditation   29
members   4
mental 75, 121
mention   1
messed   21
method   85
methods   125
mission 22
Monitoring   17
monitors   65
monthly   93
morning   70
mud-bath   14
multiple   43, 97, 128
myself 59
natural 30, 72, 74, 81, 108, 140, 144, 146
naturally   112

Printed in Germany
by Amazon Distribution
GmbH, Leipzig